The Best Keto Snack Recipes

Tasty and Easy Snack Recipes for Beginners

Shelby R. Henderson

Sommario

Introduction

Are you searching for a very easy means to cook healthy meals in the convenience of your own home? Are you looking for basic kitchen area devices that will assist you prepare some rich and also tasty dishes for you and your loved ones? Well, if that holds true, after that this is the very best overview you can utilize. This cooking guide offers to you the very best and also most ingenious cooking tool readily available these days. We're talking about the instant pot This original and beneficial pot has gotten numerous fans around the world due to the fact that it's so easy to use as well as due to the fact that it can help you cook numerous tasty dishes. You can prepare simple breakfasts, lunch recipes, treats, appetisers, side dishes, fish and fish and shellfish, meat, fowl, veggie and also treat dishes instantaneous pot. This brings us to the second part of this overview. This journal concentrates on making use of the instantaneous pot to make the most effective Ketogenic dishes. The Ketogenic diet is much more than a straightforward weight-loss program. It's a way of living that will certainly enhance your health as well as the way you look. This low-carb and high-fat diet will get your body to a state of ketosis. The diet aid you generate more ketones as well as therefore it will certainly improve your metabolism and your energy levels.

The Ketogenic diet regimen will certainly show its numerous

benefits in a matter of minutes and it will help you look much better.

Bread Twists

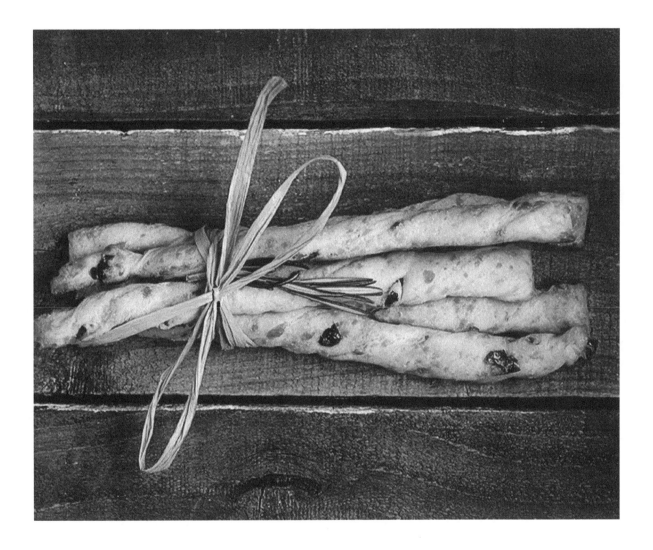

Preparation time: 15 minutes

Cooking time: 20 minutes

Servings: 7

Ingredients:

- 4 tablespoons almond flour

- 4 tablespoons coconut flour

- ¼ teaspoon salt

- ½ teaspoon baking powder

- 1 teaspoon apple cider vinegar

- 1 tablespoon butter

- ¾ cup Cheddar cheese, shredded

- 1 egg, beaten

- 1 tablespoon water

- 1 cup water, for cooking

Directions:

In the mixing bowl combine together butter and Cheddar cheese. Place the mixture in the microwave and heat it up for 30 seconds. Stir the mixture until smooth. In the separated bowl combine together almond flour, coconut flour, salt, baking powder, apple cider vinegar, and egg. When the mixture is smooth, add cheese mixture and knead the dough. After this, roll up the dough and cut it into the triangles. Twist every triangle. Pour water and insert the steamer rack in the instant pot. Line the rack with baking paper. Arrange the twists in the rack in one layer and brush with 1 tablespoon of water. Then close the lid and cook the meal for 20 minutes on manual mode (high pressure). Then make a quick pressure release and remove the twists from the instant pot.

Nutrition: calories 114, fat 8.6, fiber 2.2, carbs 4.1, protein 5.3

Italian Asparagus

Preparation time: 4 minutes

Cooking time: 4 minutes

Servings: 4

Ingredients:

- 1 cup water

- 1 pound asparagus, trimmed

- ½ tablespoon Italian seasoning

- A pinch of salt and black pepper

- 1 tablespoon cilantro, chopped

- 1 tablespoon lemon juice

- 1 teaspoon olive oil

Directions:

Put the water in your instant pot, add steamer basket, add the asparagus, put the lid on and cook on High for 4 minutes. Release the pressure fast for 4 minutes, transfer the asparagus to a bowl, add the rest of the ingredients, toss, arrange everything on a platter and serve.

Nutrition: calories 39, fat 2.1, fiber 1.1, carbs 1.3, protein 2.5

Cheese Chips

Preparation time: 5 minutes

Cooking time: 30 minutes

Servings: 5

Ingredients:

- •5 Cheddar cheese slices

Directions:

Line the instant pot with baking paper. Then place Cheddar cheese slices inside in one layer (put 2 Cheddar slices). The close the lid and cook cheese chips for 15 minutes on sauté mode or until the chips are dry (it depends on your instant pot type). When the time is over, open the lid and remove the cheese chips with baking paper. Cool the chips and then remove them from the baking paper with the help of the metal spatula. Repeat the same steps with remaining cheese slices.

Nutrition: calories 113, fat 9.3, fiber 0, carbs 0.4, protein 7

Fennel and Leeks Platter

Preparation time: 5 minutes

Cooking time: 8 minutes

Servings: 4

Ingredients:

- 4 leeks, roughly sliced

- 2 fennel bulbs, halved

- 1 tablespoon smoked paprika

- 1 teaspoon chili sauce

- A pinch of salt and black pepper

- 1 tablespoon ghee, melted

- ½ cup chicken stock

Directions:

In your instant pot, combine the leeks with the fennel, salt, pepper and the stock, put the lid on and cook on High for 8 minutes. Release the pressure fast for 5 minutes, arrange the leeks and fennel on a platter, sprinkle the paprika on top, drizzle the chili sauce and the ghee and serve as an appetizer.

Nutrition: calories 124, fat 4, fiber 2.1, carbs 3.3, protein 3.2

Butter Coffee

Preparation time: 10 minutes

Cooking time: 10 minutes

Servings: 2

Ingredients:

- 2 teaspoons instant coffee

- 2 tablespoons butter

- 1 cup of water

- ¼ cup heavy cream

Directions:

Pour water in the instant pot and bring it to boil on sauté mode. Then add instant coffee and stir it until coffee is dissolved. Then add butter and switch off the instant pot. Let the butter melts. Then pour the cooked butter coffee in the serving cups.

Nutrition: calories 154, fat 17.1, fiber 0, carbs 0.4, protein 0.4

Nutmeg Endives

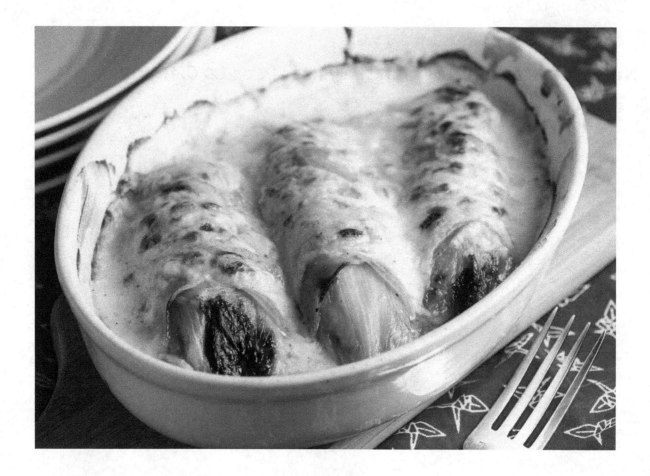

Preparation time: 10 minutes

Cooking time: 10 minutes

Servings: 4

Ingredients:

- 4 endives, trimmed and halved

- 1 cup water

- Salt and black pepper to the taste

- 2 tablespoons olive oil

- 1 teaspoon nutmeg, ground

- 1 tablespoon chives, chopped

Directions:

Add the water to your instant pot, add steamer basket, add the endives inside, put the lid on and cook on High for 10 minutes. Release the pressure naturally for 10 minutes, arrange the endives on a platter, drizzle the oil, season with salt, pepper and nutmeg, sprinkle the chives at the end and serve as an appetizer.

Nutrition: calories 63, fat 7.2, fiber 0.1, carbs 0.3, protein 0.1

Pumpkin Spices Latte

Preparation time: 10 minutes

Cooking time: 10 minutes

Servings: 2

Ingredients:

- ½ cup of coconut milk

- ¼ cup of water

- 2 teaspoons instant coffee

- 1 teaspoon pumpkin spices

- 1 teaspoon pumpkin puree

Directions:

Pour water in the instant pot. Add instant coffee and stir the liquid until it is dissolved. Then set sauté mode and bring the liquid to boil (it will take appx.3-5 minutes). Add pumpkin spices and pumpkin puree. Saute the liquid for 2 minutes more. Meanwhile, whisk the coconut milk with the help of the hand whisker until you get big foam. Pour hot coffee in the serving cups. Add coconut milk with foam.

Nutrition: calories 142, fat 14.4, fiber 1.5, carbs 4.1, protein 1.5

Thyme Eggplants and Celery Spread

Preparation time: 10 minutes

Cooking time: 12 minutes

Servings: 4

Ingredients:

- 2 pounds eggplant, roughly chopped

- A pinch of salt and black pepper

- 2 celery stalks, chopped

- 2 tablespoons olive oil

- 4 garlic cloves, minced

- ½ cup veggie stock

- 2 tablespoons lime juice

- 1 bunch thyme, chopped

Directions:

Set your instant pot on sauté mode, add the oil, heat it up, add the celery stalks and the garlic and sauté for 2 minutes. Add the rest of the ingredients, put the lid on and cook on High for 10 minutes. Release the pressure naturally for 10 minutes, blend the mix using an immersion blender, divide into cups and serve as a spread.

Nutrition: calories 123, fat 7.4, fiber 1.8, carbs 3.7, protein 2.5

Salty Nuts Mix

Preparation time: 10 minutes

Cooking time: 7 minutes

Servings: 5

Ingredients:

- 1 teaspoon coconut aminos

- 1 teaspoon coconut oil

- ½ teaspoon sesame oil

- ¼ teaspoon chili powder

- 1 teaspoon salt

- 2 tablespoons walnuts

- 5 pecans

- 1 tablespoon pistachios

- 1 tablespoon cashew

Directions:

Place coconut oil and sesame oil in the instant pot. Heat up the oils on sauté mode for 1 minute. Then add coconut aminos, chili powder, walnuts, pecans, pistachios, and cashew. Mix up the nuts and cook them for 5 minutes. Stir the nuts every 1 minute. Add salt and mix up the mixture. Transfer the nut mix in the paper bag.

Nutrition: calories 144, fat 14.4, fiber 1.9, carbs 3.3, protein 2.7

Shrimp and Okra Bowls

Preparation time: 10 minutes

Cooking time: 12 minutes

Servings: 4

Ingredients:

- 1 pound okra, trimmed

- ½ pound shrimp, peeled and deveined

- A pinch of salt and black pepper

- 2 tablespoons olive oil

- 1 cup tomato passata, chopped

- 1 tablespoon cilantro, chopped

Directions:

In your instant pot, combine the okra with the shrimp and the rest of the ingredients, put the lid on and cook on High for 12 minutes. Release the pressure fast for 5 minutes, divide the mix into bowls and serve as an appetizer.

Nutrition: calories 188, fat 8.3, fiber 4.6, carbs 6.1, protein 15.6

Heart of Palm Dip

Preparation time: 10 minutes

Cooking time: 8 minutes

Servings: 8

Ingredients:

- 1-pound heart of palm, chopped

- 1 garlic clove, diced

- 1 tablespoon avocado oil

- 1 teaspoon lemon juice

- ½ teaspoon salt

- ¼ teaspoon ground black pepper

- ¼ teaspoon fennel seeds

- ¼ cup heavy cream

- 1 oz Provolone cheese, grated

Directions:

Pour avocado oil in the instant pot and heat it up. Add diced garlic, ground black pepper, and fennel seeds. Cook the ingredients for 2 minutes or until they become aromatic. Meanwhile, put the heart of palms in the blender. Add lemon juice. Blend the mixture until smooth. Add heavy cream and cheese in the hot oil mixture and bring it to boil. Remove the liquid from the heat and add it in the blender heart of palm. Stir well. Store the dip in the fridge for up to 8 hours.

Nutrition: calories 45, fat 2.9, fiber 1.5, carbs 3.1, protein 2.5

Mushrooms Salsa

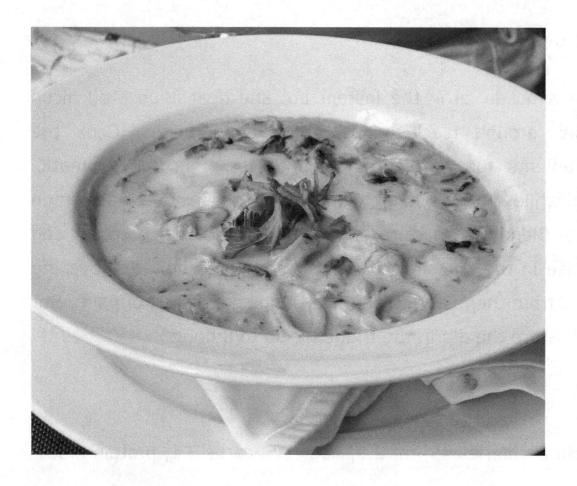

Preparation time: 10 minutes

Cooking time: 10 minutes

Servings: 4

Ingredients:

- 1 pound white mushrooms, halved

- A pinch of salt and black pepper

- 1 tablespoon ghee, melted

- ¼ cup chicken stock

- 1 tablespoon rosemary, chopped

- 1 tablespoon basil, chopped

- 1 tablespoon oregano, chopped

- 2 tomatoes, cubed

- 1 avocado, peeled, pitted and cubed

Directions:

In your instant pot, combine the mushrooms with salt, pepper and the rest of the ingredients, put the lid on and cook on High for 10 minutes. Release the pressure naturally for 10 minutes, divide the salsa into bowls and serve as an appetizer.

Nutrition: calories 173, fat 13.7, fiber 6.2, carbs 7.7, protein 5.3

Taco Shells

Preparation time: 15 minutes

Cooking time: 50 minutes

Servings:4

Ingredients:

- •4 lettuce leaves

- •¼ cup radish, chopped

- •10 oz beef sirloin

- •½ teaspoon dried cilantro

- •½ teaspoon salt

- •½ teaspoon dried oregano

- •1 teaspoon taco seasoning

- •1 teaspoon green chile

- ½ cup chicken broth

- 1 teaspoon ground paprika

- 1 teaspoon cream cheese

Directions:

Put beef sirloin, dried cilantro, salt, oregano, taco seasonings, green chile, ground paprika, and chicken broth in the instant pot. Close the lid and cook meat on stew/meat mode for 50 minutes. When the time is over, remove the meat from the instant pot and shred it. Then mix up together 3 tablespoons chicken broth from instant pot and cream cheese. Stir the liquid in the shredded meat and stir well. Then fill the lettuce leaves with shredded beef.

Nutrition: calories 146, fat 5, fiber 0.4, carbs 1.5, protein 22.4

Cheesy Mushroom and Tomato Salad

Preparation time: 10 minutes

Cooking time: 10 minutes

Servings: 4

Ingredients:

- 4 tomatoes, cubed

- ½ cup veggie stock

- A pinch of salt and black pepper

- 1 tablespoon ghee, melted

- 1 pound mushrooms, halved

- 1 cup mozzarella, shredded

- 1 tablespoon parsley, chopped

Directions:

Set your instant pot on sauté mode, add the ghee, heat it up, add the mushrooms, stir and sauté for 2 minutes. Add the rest of the ingredients except the mozzarella and toss. Sprinkle the mozzarella on top, put the lid on and cook on High for 8 minutes. Release the pressure naturally for 10 minutes, divide the mix into bowls and serve as an appetizer.

Nutrition: calories 95, fat 5, fiber 2.3, carbs 4.7, protein 6.7

Mini Margharita Pizzas in Mushroom Caps

Preparation time: 15 minutes

Cooking time: 10 minutes

Servings:4

Ingredients:

- 4 Portobello mushroom caps

- 1/3 cup Mozzarella, shredded

- 1 teaspoon fresh basil, chopped

- 1 teaspoon cream cheese

- ¼ teaspoon dried oregano

- 1 teaspoon tomato sauce

- 1 cup water, for cooking

Directions:

Pour water and insert the trivet in the instant pot. Then mix up together shredded Mozzarella, basil, cream cheese, and dried oregano. Fill the mushroom caps with the Mozzarella mixture. Top every Portobello cap with tomato sauce and transfer in the trivet. Close the lid and cook pizzas for 10 minutes on manual mode (high pressure). When the time is over, make a quick pressure release and transfer the cooked Margharita pizzas on the plate.

Nutrition: calories 10, fat 0.7, fiber 0.1, carbs 0.3, protein 0.8

Olives Spread

Preparation time: 10 minutes

Cooking time: 15 minutes

Servings: 4

Ingredients:

- 2 cups black olives, pitted and haled

- 2 garlic cloves, minced

- 1 tablespoon lemon juice

- 1 tablespoon olive oil

- A pinch of salt and black pepper

- 1 tablespoon parsley, chopped

- ¼ cup chicken stock

Directions:

In your instant pot, combine the black olives with the stock, salt and the rest of the ingredients, put the lid on and cook on High for 10 minutes. Release the pressure naturally for 10 minutes, blend the mix using an immersion blender, divide into bowls and serve as a party spread.

Nutrition: calories 111, fat 10.8, fiber 2.2, carbs 4.9, protein 0.8

Keto Guacamole Deviled Eggs

Preparation time: 20 minutes

Cooking time: 5 minutes

Servings:6

Ingredients:

- 6 eggs

- 1 avocado, pitted, peeled

- 2 tablespoons lemon juice

- ¼ teaspoon salt

- 1 tablespoon cream cheese

- 1 teaspoon chives, chopped

- 1 cup water, for cooking

Directions:

Pour water and insert the steamer rack in the instant pot. Place the eggs in the trivet and close the lid. Cook them on Manual (high pressure) for 5 minutes. Then allow the natural pressure release for 5 minutes. Cool the eggs in ice water and peel. Then cut them into halves and remove the egg yolks. Place the egg yolks in the bowl. Chop the avocado and add it in the egg yolks. Smash the mixture with the fork until smooth. Then add cream cheese, salt, and lemon juice. Mix up well and add chives. Stir the guacamole mixture little. Fill the egg whites with guacamole mass.

Nutrition: calories 138, fat 11.5, fiber 2.3, carbs 3.4, protein 6.4

Basil Stuffed Bell Peppers

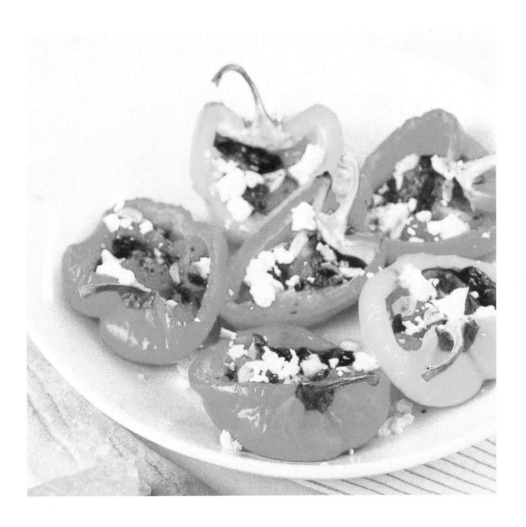

Preparation time: 10 minutes

Cooking time: 15 minutes

Servings: 4

Ingredients:

- 4 red bell peppers, tops cut off and deseeded

- 2 tablespoons parsley, chopped

- 2 cups basil, chopped

- ¼ cup mozzarella, shredded

- 1 tablespoon garlic, minced

- 2 teaspoons lemon juice

- 1 cup baby spinach, torn

- 2 cups water

Directions:

In a bowl, mix all the ingredients except the water and the peppers, stir well and stuff the peppers with this mix. Add the water to your instant pot, add the trivet inside, arrange the bell peppers in the pot, put the lid on and cook on High for 15 minutes. Release the pressure naturally for 10 minutes, arrange the peppers on a platter and serve as an appetizer.

Nutrition: calories 52, fat 4.8, fiber 2.4, carbs 3.6, protein 2.5

Hot Tempeh

Preparation time: 10 minutes

Cooking time: 9 minutes

Servings:4

Ingredients:

- •8 oz tempeh

- •1 teaspoon chili powder

- •¼ teaspoon ground paprika

- •¼ teaspoon ground turmeric

- •1 teaspoon avocado oil

Directions:

Cut the tempeh into 4 servings. After this, in the shallow bowl mix up together chili powder, ground paprika, turmeric, and avocado oil. Rub the tempeh with chili powder mixture from each side. Preheat the instant pot on sauté mode for 3 minutes. Then add tempeh and cook it for 3 minutes from each side.

Nutrition: calories 114, fat 6.4, fiber 0.4, carbs 5.9, protein 10.6

Mussels Salad

Preparation time: 10 minutes

Cooking time: 6 minutes

Servings: 4

Ingredients:

- 1 pound mussels, scrubbed

- 2 cups baby spinach

- ½ cup chicken stock

- 1 tablespoon balsamic vinegar

- 2 scallions, chopped

- ½ teaspoon olive oil

- ½ teaspoon chili powder

- ½ teaspoon oregano, chopped

- A pinch of salt and black pepper

Directions:

In your instant pot, mix the mussels with the stock, salt and pepper, put the lid on and cook on High for 6 minutes. Release the pressure naturally for 10 minutes, transfer the mussels to a bowl, add the rest of the ingredients, toss, and serve as an appetizer.

Nutrition: calories 112, fat 3.4, fiber 0.7, carbs 1.7, protein 14.1

Garlic Aioli

Preparation time: 15 minutes

Cooking time: 4 minutes

Servings:4

Ingredients:

- •4 garlic cloves, peeled

- •1 teaspoon lime juice

- •1 teaspoon mustard

- •½ cup heavy cream

- •¼ teaspoon ground black pepper

- •¼ teaspoon salt

- •1 cup water, for cooking

Directions:

Wrap the garlic in the foil. Then pour water and insert the steamer rack in the instant pot. Place the wrapped garlic in the rack and close the lid. Cook it on manual (high pressure) for 4 minutes. Then allow the natural pressure release for 5 minutes and open the lid. Remove the garlic from the foil and transfer it in the bowl. Smash it with the help of the fork until you get puree texture. After this, add lime juice, mustard, ground black pepper, salt. Stir the mixture. Whip the heavy cream. Then combine together whipped cream and garlic mixture. Store the meal in the fridge for up to 4 days.

Nutrition: calories 61, fat 5.8, fiber 0.2, carbs 2, protein 0.7

Oregano Beef Bites

Preparation time: 10 minutes

Cooking time: 15 minutes

Servings: 4

Ingredients:

- 1 tablespoon lime juice

- 2 tablespoons avocado oil

- 1 pound beef stew meat, cubed

- 2 garlic cloves, minced

- 1 tablespoon smoked paprika

- 1 tablespoon oregano, chopped

- 1 tablespoon lime zest, grated

- 1 cup beef stock

Directions:

Set the instant pot on Sauté mode, add the oil, heat it up, add the meat and brown for 5 minutes. Add the rest of the ingredients, put the lid on and cook on High for 10 minutes. Release the pressure naturally for 10 minutes, arrange the beef bites on a platter and serve.

Nutrition: calories 236, fat 8.4, fiber 1.6, carbs 2.8, protein 34.5

Pesto Wings

Preparation time: 10 minutes

Cooking time: 15 minutes

Servings:6

Ingredients:

- •6 chicken wings

- •1 teaspoon ground paprika

- •1 teaspoon butter

- •4 teaspoons pesto sauce

- •2 tablespoons cream cheese

Directions:

Rub the chicken wings with ground paprika. Toss butter in the instant pot and heat it up on sauté mode. When the butter is melted, place the chicken wings inside (in one layer) and cook them for 3 minutes from each side or until you get light brown color. Then add pesto sauce and cream cheese. Coat the chicken wings in the mixture well, bring to boil, and close the lid. Saute the wings for 4 minutes.

Nutrition: calories 127, fat 9.6, fiber 0.3, carbs 3.7, protein 6.4

Watercress and Zucchini Salsa

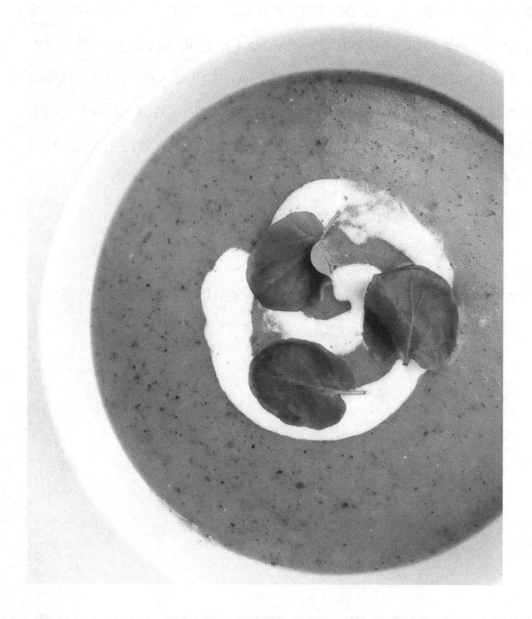

Preparation time: 5 minutes

Cooking time: 12 minutes

Servings: 4

Ingredients:

- 1 bunch watercress, trimmed

- Juice of 1 lime

- ¼ cup chicken stock

- 2 teaspoons thyme, dried

- 2 tablespoons avocado oil

- 1 cup tomato, cubed

- 1 avocado, peeled, pitted and cubed

- 2 zucchinis, cubed

- 2 spring onions, chopped

- 3 garlic cloves, minced

- ¼ cup cilantro, chopped

- 1 tablespoon balsamic vinegar

Directions:

Set the instant pot on Sauté mode, add the oil, heat it up, add the garlic and sauté for 2 minutes. Add the rest of the ingredients, put the lid on and cook on High for 10 minutes. Release the pressure fast for 5 minutes, divide the salsa into cups and serve as an appetizer.

Nutrition: calories 144, fat 11.1, fiber 4.4, carbs 5.3, protein 3

Bacon Avocado Bombs

Preparation time: 20 minutes

Cooking time: 10 minutes

Servings:8

Ingredients:

- 1 avocado, pitted, peeled

- 3 eggs

- 2 bacon slices, chopped

- 4 tablespoons cream cheese

- ½ teaspoon green onion, minced

- 1 cup water, for cooking

Directions:

Pour water and insert the steamer rack in the instant pot. Place the egg on the rack and close the lid. Cook them for 5 minutes on steam mode. When the time is over, allow the natural pressure release for 5 minutes more. Then cool the eggs in ice water and peel. Clean the instant pot and remove the steamer rack. Put the chopped bacon slices in the instant pot and cook them on sauté mode for minutes or until crunchy. Stir the bacon every minute. Meanwhile, chop the avocado and eggs into tiny pieces and place the ingredients in the big bowl. Add minced green onion and cream cheese. With the help of the fork mix up the mixture and smash it gently (we don't need smooth texture).Then add cooked bacon and stir until homogenous. With the help of the scopper make the balls and refrigerate them for 10-15 minutes. Store the bacon avocado bombs in the fridge in the closed vessel for up to 8 days.

Nutrition: calories 118, fat 10.3, fiber 1.7, carbs 2.5, protein 4.7

Basil Shallots and Peppers Dip

Preparation time: 5 minutes

Cooking time: 15 minutes

Servings: 2

Ingredients:

- ½ cup lemon juice

- 3 shallots, minced

- ½ teaspoon hot sauce

- 1 tablespoon balsamic vinegar

- 1 and ½ pounds mixed peppers, roughly chopped

- ¼ cup chicken stock

- 1 tablespoon olive oil

- 2 tablespoons basil, chopped

Directions:

Set the instant pot on Sauté mode, add the oil, heat it up, add the shallots and sauté for 2 minutes. Add the rest of the ingredients, put the lid on and cook on High for 13 minutes. Release the pressure fast for 5 minutes, blend the mix using an immersion blender, divide into bowls and serve.

Nutrition: calories 78, fat 7.6, fiber 0.3, carbs 1.5, protein 0.7

Bacon Sushi

Preparation time: 15 minutes

Cooking time: 4 minutes

Servings:6

Ingredients:

- •6 bacon slices

- •1 cucumber

- •3 teaspoons cream cheese

- •¼ teaspoon ground black pepper

- •¼ teaspoon salt

- •¼ teaspoon dried thyme

- •½ teaspoon coconut oil

Directions:

Sprinkle the bacon slices with dried thyme, salt, and ground black pepper. Put coconut oil in the instant pot. Melt it on sauté mode. Then arrange the bacon in one layer. Cook it for 1 minute and flip on another side. Cook the bacon for 1 minute more. Then transfer the bacon on the paper towel and dry well. Place the dried bacon on the sushi mat in the shape of the net. Then spread the bacon net with cream cheese. Cut the cucumber into the sticks. Place the cucumber sticks over the cream cheese. Roll the bacon in the shape of sushi and cut into 6 servings.

Nutrition: calories 120, fat 9, fiber 0.3, carbs 2.2, protein 7.5

Olives and Spinach Dip

Preparation time: 5 minutes

Cooking time: 10 minutes

Servings: 4

Ingredients:

- 4 cups baby spinach

- ½ cup coconut cream

- A pinch of salt and black pepper

- 2 tablespoons avocado oil

- 4 garlic cloves, roasted and minced

- 2 tablespoons lime juice

- 1 tablespoon chives, chopped

- 1 cup kalamata olives, pitted and halved

Directions:

In your instant pot, combine all the ingredients except the chives, put the lid on and cook on High for 10 minutes. Release the pressure fast for 5 minutes, blend the mix using an immersion blender, add chives, stir, divide into bowls and serve as a party dip.

Nutrition: calories 129, fat 11.8, fiber 2.8, carbs 6.3, protein 2.1

Ranch Poppers

Preparation time: 15 minutes

Cooking time: 4 minute

Servings:8

Ingredients:

- ½ cup ground chicken

- ¼ cup zucchini, grated

- 1 teaspoon dried cilantro

- ¼ teaspoon garlic powder

- 1 teaspoon almond flour

- 1 teaspoon olive oil

- ½ teaspoon salt

Directions:

Mix up together ground chicken, grated zucchini, cilantro, garlic powder, and almond flour. Add salt and stir the mas until homogenous. Make the small balls (poppers) with the help of the fingertips. Pour olive oil in the instant pot. Arrange the ranch poppers in the instant pot and cook them for 1.5 minutes from each side.

Nutrition: calories 43, fat 3, fiber 0.4, carbs 0.9, protein 3.3

Mint Salmon and Radish Salad

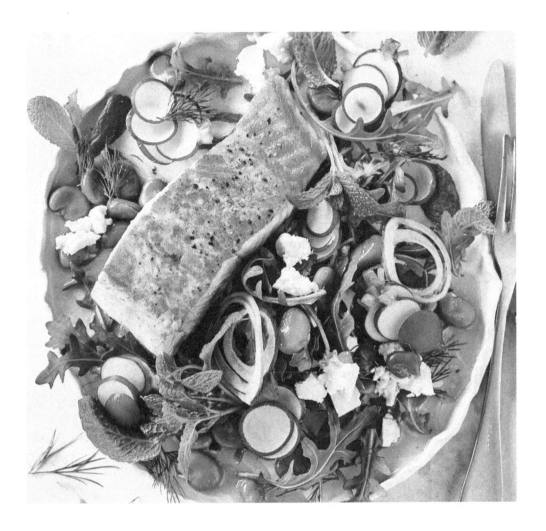

Preparation time: 10 minutes

Cooking time: 15 minutes

Servings: 4

Ingredients:

- 1 pound salmon fillets, boneless, skinless and cubed

- 2 cups red radishes, sliced

- 1 shallot, sliced

- ½ tablespoons avocado oil

- 2 tablespoons mint leaves, chopped

- ½ cup coconut cream

- A pinch of salt and black pepper

Directions:

Set the instant pot on Sauté mode, add the oil, heat it up, add the shallot and sauté for 2 minutes. Add the salmon and cook for 2 minutes more. Add the rest of the ingredients, put the lid on and cook on High for 10 minutes. Release the pressure naturally for 10 minutes, divide the mix into bowls and serve as an appetizer.

Nutrition: calories 232, fat 14.5, fiber 1.9, carbs 4, protein 23.2

Keto Taquitos

Preparation time: 15 minutes

Cooking time: 20 minutes

Servings:6

Ingredients:

- •3 low carb tortillas

- •¼ teaspoon onion powder

- •¼ cup Cheddar cheese, shredded

- •5 oz chicken breast, skinless, boneless

- •½ teaspoon ground black pepper

- •¼ teaspoon salt

- •½ teaspoon cayenne pepper

- •1 teaspoon butter

●1 cup water, for cooking

Directions:

Rub the chicken breast with salt, cayenne pepper, and ground black pepper. Pour water and insert the steamer rack in the instant pot. Arrange the chicken in the steamer rack and close the lid. Cook it on manual mode (high pressure) for 15 minutes. Then make a quick pressure release and transfer the chicken on the chopping board. Shred the chicken. Place the shredded chicken in the mixing bowl. Add onion powder and shredded Cheddar cheese. Mix up the mixture well. Then spread tortillas with chicken mixture and roll. Clean the instant pot and remove the rack. Toss the butter in the instant pot, melt it on sauté mode. Arrange the rolled tortillas in the instant pot in one layer. Cook them for 2 minutes from each side. When taquitos are cooked, remove them from the instant pot and cut into 6 servings.

Nutrition: calories 93, fat 3.8, fiber 3.6, carbs 6.3, protein 7.7

Red Chard Spread

Preparation time: 10 minutes

Cooking time: 15 minutes

Servings: 4

Ingredients:

- 1 pound red chard

- 1 cup spring onions, chopped

- 1 cup veggie stock

- 1 tablespoon sweet paprika

- 1 tablespoon lime juice

- 2 tablespoons olive oil

- 2 garlic cloves, minced

- ½ cup coconut cream

- 1 tablespoon chives, chopped

Directions:

In your instant pot, combine chard with the rest of the ingredients except the cream and the chives, put the lid on and cook on High for 15 minutes. Release the pressure naturally for 10 minutes, add the cream, blend everything using an immersion blender, divide into bowls, sprinkle the chives on top and serve.

Nutrition: calories 144, fat 14.4, fiber 2, carbs 5, protein 1.5

Chicken Celery Boats

Preparation time: 10 minutes

Cooking time: 10 minutes

Servings:2

Ingredients:

- •2 celery stalks

- •3 oz chicken fillet

- •¼ teaspoon minced garlic

- •¼ teaspoon salt

- •1 teaspoon cream cheese

- •1 cup water, for cooking

Directions:

Pour water and insert the steamer rack in the instant pot. Put the chicken on the rack and close the lid. Cook it on manual mode (high pressure) for 10 minutes. Then make a quick pressure release and remove the chicken from the instant pot. Shred the chicken and mix it up with minced garlic, salt, and cream cheese. Fill the celery stalks with chicken mixture.

Nutrition: calories 90, fat 3.8, fiber 0.3, carbs 0.7, protein 12.6

Salmon and Swiss Chard Salad

Preparation time: 10 minutes

Cooking time: 15 minutes

Servings: 4

Ingredients:

- 1 teaspoon olive oil

- 1 pound salmon fillets, boneless, skinless and cubed

- A pinch of salt and black pepper

- ¼ pound Swiss chard, torn

- 1 tablespoon rosemary, chopped

- 1 tablespoon lime juice

- 1 spring onion, chopped

- ¼ cup chicken stock

Directions:

Set the instant pot on Sauté mode, add the oil, heat it up, add the spring onion and sauté for 2 minutes. Add the salmon and cook for 2 minutes on each side. Add the rest of the ingredients, put the lid on and cook on High for 10 minutes. Release the pressure naturally for 10 minutes, divide the mix into bowls and serve as an appetizer.

Nutrition: calories 170, fat 8.4, fiber 0.9, carbs 1.9, protein 22.7

Keto Nachos

Preparation time: 10 minutes

Cooking time: 27 minutes

Servings:2

Ingredients:

- ½ cup mini bell peppers

- ½ cup ground beef

- ¼ teaspoon chili powder

- ¼ teaspoon ground cumin

- ¼ teaspoon dried thyme

- ¼ teaspoon onion powder

- ¼ teaspoon garlic powder

- 2 oz Provolone cheese, grated

- 1 teaspoon coconut oil

Directions:

Put coconut oil in the instant pot and preheat it on sauté mode until it is melted. Then add ground beef, chili powder, ground cumin, thyme, onion powder, and garlic powder. Mix up the mixture well with the help of a spatula and cook on sauté mode for 15 minutes. Stir it from time to time. When the time is over, cut the mini bell peppers into halves and place them in the instant pot. Cook the keto nachos for 10 minutes more. The cooked bell peppers shouldn't be soft.

Nutrition: calories 213, fat 14, fiber 1.2, carbs 6.5, protein 15

Basil Peppers Salsa

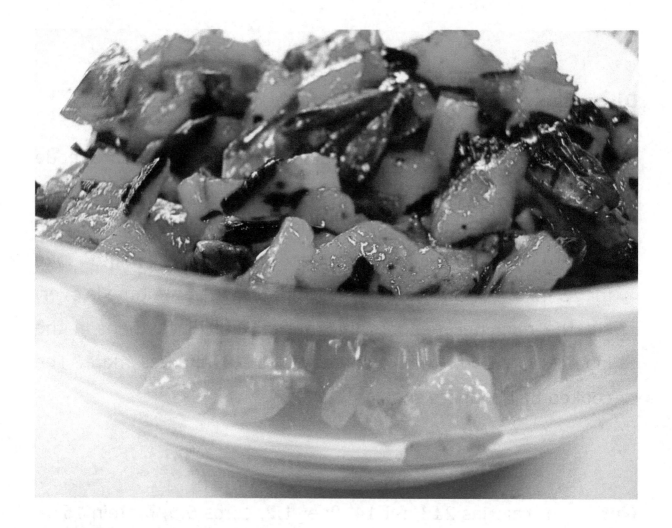

Preparation time: 10 minutes

Cooking time: 12 minutes

Servings: 4

Ingredients:

- 1 and ½ pounds mixed bell peppers, cut into strips

- 2 tablespoons parsley, chopped

- 2 tablespoons basil, chopped

- 2 teaspoons lime juice

- 1 tablespoon avocado oil

- ½ cup tomato passata

- 2 tomatoes, cubed

- 1 avocado, peeled, pitted and cubed

- A pinch of salt and black pepper

Directions:

In your instant pot, combine all the ingredients, put the lid on and cook o High for 12 minutes. Release the pressure naturally for 10 minutes, transfer the mix to small bowls, toss and serve as an appetizer.

Nutrition: calories 127, fat 10.5, fiber 4.8, carbs 7.8, protein 2

Edamame Hummus

Preparation time: 15 minutes

Cooking time: 5 minutes

Servings:8

Ingredients:

- •1 ½ cup edamame beans, shelled

- •1 teaspoon salt

- •½ teaspoon harissa

- •1 garlic clove, peeled

- •4 tablespoons olive oil

- •1 tablespoon lemon juice

- •1 avocado, pitted, peeled, chopped

- •1 cup water, for cooking

Directions:

Pour water in the instant pot. Add edamame beans and garlic, and close the lid. Cook the beans on manual mode (high pressure) for 2 minutes. Then make a quick pressure release and open the lid. Transfer the edamame beans and garlic in the blender. Add 1/3 cup of water from the instant pot. Then add harissa, salt, lemon juice, and avocado. Blend the mixture until it is smooth and soft. Add more water if the texture of the hummus is very thick. Then add olive oil and pulse the hummus for 10 seconds. Transfer the cooked edamame hummus in the serving bowl.

Nutrition: calories 99, fat 9, fiber 2.2, carbs 3.5, protein 2.5

Pesto Chicken Salad

Preparation time: 10 minutes

Cooking time: 20 minutes

Servings: 4

Ingredients:

- 1 pound chicken breast, skinless, boneless and cubed

- 2 tablespoons basil pesto

- 2 tablespoons olive oil

- 2 spring onions, chopped

- 2 tablespoons garlic, chopped

- 1 cup chicken stock

- 1 cup tomatoes, crushed

- 1 tablespoon oregano, chopped

Directions:

Set your instant pot on Sauté mode, add the oil, heat it up, add the chicken and the onions and brown for 5 minutes. Add the rest of the ingredients except the basil, put the lid on and cook on High for 15 minutes. Release the pressure naturally for 10 minutes, divide the mix into bowls and serve right away.

Nutrition: calories 212, fat 10.2, fiber 1.3, carbs 4.6, protein 25.2

Crab Spread

Preparation time: 10 minutes

Cooking time: 4 minutes

Servings:6

Ingredients:

- ½ cup cauliflower, chopped

- 10 oz crab meat

- 1 teaspoon minced garlic

- ½ cup cream cheese

- 1 tablespoon fresh cilantro, chopped

- 1 cup water, for cooking

Directions:

Place crab meat and cauliflower in the instant pot. Add water and close the lid. Cook the ingredients for 4 minutes on manual mode (high pressure). Then remove the cooked cauliflower and crab meat from the instant pot. Chop the crab meat into small pieces. Then smash the cauliflower with the help of the fork. The smashed mixture shouldn't be smooth. Mix up together cauliflower, crab meat, minced garlic, cream cheese, and cilantro. Mix up the spread well and store it in the fridge for up to 3 days.

Nutrition: calories 112, fat 7.6, fiber 0.2, carbs 2, protein 7.6

Cabbage and Spinach Slaw

Preparation time: 10 minutes

Cooking time: 15 minutes

Servings: 4

Ingredients:

- 2 cups red cabbage, shredded

- 1 tablespoon avocado mayonnaise

- 1 spring onion, chopped

- 1 pound baby spinach

- ½ cup chicken stock

- 1 teaspoon chili powder

- 1 tablespoon sweet paprika

- 1 tablespoon chives, chopped

- 1 tablespoon avocado oil

Directions:

Set instant pot on Sauté mode, add the oil, heat it up, add the onion and cook for 2 minutes. Add the rest of the ingredients except the spinach, avocado mayonnaise and the chives, put the lid on and cook on High for 12 minutes. Release the pressure naturally for 10 minutes, transfer the mix to a bowl, add the remaining ingredients, toss and serve as an appetizer.

Nutrition: calories 72, fat 3.8, fiber 1.2, carbs 2.6, protein 4.3

Bacon-Wrapped Shrimps

Preparation time: 15 minutes

Cooking time: 8 minutes

Servings:4

Ingredients:

- •4 king shrimps, peeled·

- •4 bacon slices

- •¼ teaspoon chili flakes

- •¼ teaspoon ground black pepper

- •¼ teaspoon salt

- •½ teaspoon avocado oil

- •1 cup water, for cooking

Directions:

Brush the instant pot bowl with avocado oil and heat it up for 2 minutes on sauté mode. Arrange the bacon slices in one layer and cook for 2 minutes from each side. Cool the cooked bacon. Clean the instant pot. Place the steamer rack and pour water in the instant pot. Place the shrimps in the mixing bowl. Add chili flakes, ground black pepper, and salt. Mix up the spices and shrimps. Then wrap every shrimp in cooked bacon. Secure them with toothpicks. Place the shrimps on the rack and close the lid. Cook the seafood for 2 minutes on manual mode (high pressure). When the time is over, make a quick pressure release.

Nutrition: calories 127, fat 8.3, fiber 0.1, carbs 0.4, protein 12.4

Cabbage, Tomato and Avocado Salsa

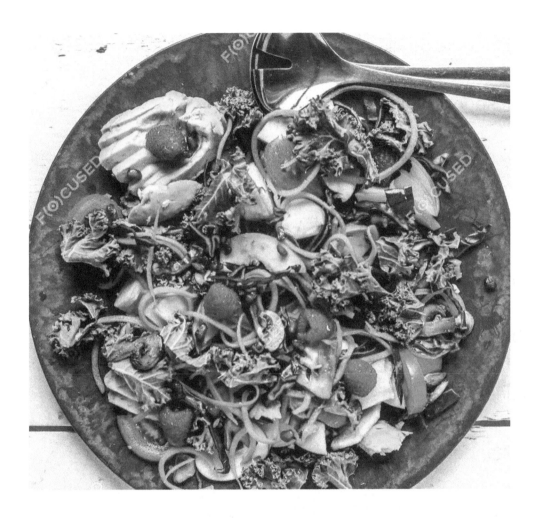

Preparation time: 5 minutes

Cooking time: 12 minutes

Servings: 4

Ingredients:

- 1 and ½ pound cherry tomatoes, cubed
- ¼ cup veggie stock
- 2 tablespoons olive oil
- ¼ cup balsamic vinegar
- 2 spring onions, chopped
- 1 red cabbage head, shredded
- 1 tablespoon basil, chopped
- 1 tablespoon parsley, chopped
- 1 tablespoon chives, chopped
- 1 avocado, peeled, pitted and cubed

Directions:

In your instant pot, combine the tomatoes the rest of the ingredients, put the lid on and cook on High for 12 minutes.

Release the pressure fast for 5 minutes, transfer the mix to small bowls and serve as an appetizer.

Nutrition: calories 254, fat 17.3, fiber 2.5, carbs 5.5, protein 5.4

Tuna Steak Skewers

Preparation time: 15 minutes

Cooking time: 5 minutes

Servings:4

Ingredients:

- •2 tuna steaks

- •¼ teaspoon salt

- •1 teaspoon ground paprika

- •¾ teaspoon dried sage

- •1 cup water, for cooking

Directions:

Chop the tuna steaks into medium cubes and sprinkle with salt, ground paprika, and dried sage. Then string the meat on the skewers. Pour water and insert the steamer rack in the instant pot. Arrange the tuna steak skewers on the rack and close the lid. Cook the snack for 5 minutes on manual mode (high pressure). Then allow the natural pressure release for 10 minutes.

Nutrition: calories 158, fat 5.4, fiber 0.3, carbs 0.4, protein 25.5

Shrimp and Mussels Salad

Preparation time: 6 minutes

Cooking time: 12 minutes

Servings: 4

Ingredients:

- 1 pound mussels, scrubbed

- ½ cup tomato passata

- ¼ cup chicken stock

- 1 pound shrimp, peeled and deveined

- 1 and ½ cups baby spinach

- 2 tablespoons olive oil

- 1 teaspoon hot paprika

- 2 teaspoons oregano, dried

- 1 tablespoon parsley, chopped

Directions:

In your instant pot, combine the mussels with the rest of the ingredients except the parsley and the spinach, put the lid on and cook on High for 10 minutes. Release the pressure fast for 6 minutes, set the pot on Sauté mode again, add the spinach and the parsley, toss, cook for 2 minutes more, divide into bowls and serve as an appetizer.

Nutrition: calories 303, fat 11.7, fiber 0.8, carbs 7.8, protein 39.3

Marinated Olives

Preparation time: 10 minutes

Cooking time: 4 minutes

Servings:7

Ingredients:

- •7 kalamata olives

- •2 tablespoons lemon juice

- •¼ teaspoon peppercorns

- •¼ teaspoon minced garlic

- •¼ teaspoon fennel seeds

- •¼ teaspoon thyme

- •1 bay leaf

- •4 tablespoons avocado oil

Directions:

Pour avocado oil in the instant pot. Add bay leaf, thyme, fennel seeds, minced garlic, peppercorns, and lemon juice. Cook the ingredients on sauté mode for 4 minutes or until it is brought to boil. Then add olives and coat them in the oil mixture well. Switch off the instant pot. Transfer the cooked olives in the glass can and let them cool to room temperature. Marinate the olives for 2-3 days in the fridge.

Nutrition: calories 18, fat 1.5, fiber 0.6, carbs 1, protein 0.2

Beef, Arugula and Olives Salad

Preparation time: 10 minutes

Cooking time: 20 minutes

Servings: 4

Ingredients:

- 1 and ½ pounds beef, cut into strips

- 2 tomatoes, cubed

- ¼ cup beef stock

- ½ cup black olives, pitted and sliced

- 1 tablespoon avocado oil

- 2 spring onions, chopped

- ½ cup cilantro chopped

- 2 cups tomatoes, chopped

- 1 tablespoon basil, chopped

- A pinch of salt and black pepper

- 1 cup baby arugula

Directions:

Set your instant pot on Sauté mode, add the oil, heat it up, add the onions and the meat and brown for 5 minutes. Add the rest of the ingredients except the arugula, put the lid on and cook on High for 15 minutes. Release the pressure naturally for 10 minutes, transfer the mix to a bowl, add the arugula, toss and serve as an appetizer.

Nutrition: calories 378, fat 16.7, fiber 2.8, carbs 7.8, protein 24.3

Chicharrones

Preparation time: 15 minutes

Cooking time: 35 minutes

Servings:4

Ingredients:

- •8 oz pork skin

- •¼ teaspoon salt

- •½ teaspoon avocado oil

- •1 cup water, for cooking

Directions:

Pour water in the instant pot. Add pork skin and close the lid. Cook it on manual mode (high pressure) for 25 minutes. Then allow the natural pressure release for 10 minutes. Remove the pork skin from the instant pot. Clean the instant pot. Chop the pork skin into small pieces and return back in the instant pot. Add oil and salt. Mix up well. Cook the meal on sauté mode for 10 minutes. Stir it from time to time to avoid burning.

Nutrition: calories 309, fat 17.8, fiber 0, carbs 0, protein 34.8

Bacon Radish And Shrimp Salad

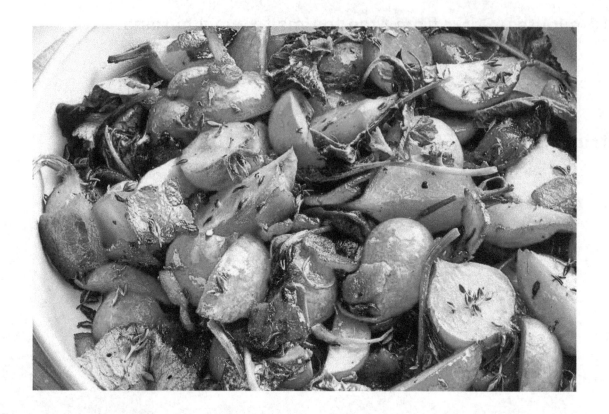

Preparation time: 5 minutes

Cooking time: 15 minutes

Servings: 4

Ingredients:

- 1 pound shrimp, peeled and deveined

- 1 shallot, chopped

- 2 cups radishes, sliced

- 1 cup bacon, cooked and crumbled

- 1 tablespoon olive oil

- 1 teaspoon sweet paprika

- 1 tablespoon oregano, chopped

- A pinch of salt and black pepper

- 1 cup veggie stock

Directions:

Set your instant pot on Sauté mode, add the oil, heat it up, add the shallot and sauté for 2 minutes. Add the rest of the ingredients except the oregano and the bacon, put the lid on and cook on High for 13 minutes. Release the pressure fast for 5 minutes, transfer the mix to small bowls, sprinkle the oregano and the bacon on top and serve as an appetizer.

Nutrition: calories 179, fat 5.7, fiber 1.6, carbs 4.5, protein 26.5

Keto Spanakopita Pie Slices

Preparation time: 20 minutes

Cooking time: 50 minutes

Servings:6

Ingredients:

- •4 tablespoons butter, softened

- •4 tablespoons coconut flour

- •4 tablespoons almond flour

- •¼ teaspoon baking powder

- •¼ teaspoon ground nutmeg

- •¼ teaspoon salt

- •3 eggs

- •1 cups fresh spinach, chopped

- 1 cup cheddar cheese, shredded

- 2 tablespoons cream cheese

- 1 cup water, for cooking

Directions:

Make the spanakopita crust: mix up together butter, coconut flour, almond flour, baking powder, ground nutmeg, and salt. Crack 1 egg inside the mixture and knead the non-sticky dough. Then line the instant pot baking pan with baking paper and place the dough inside. Flatten it in the shape of the pie crust. In the mixing bowl combine together cream cheese, shredded Cheddar cheese, spinach, and cracked remaining eggs. Stir it well. Place the mixture over the pie crust and flatten it. Cover the surface of spanakopita with baking paper. Pour water and insert the rack in the instant pot. Place the pan with spanakopita in the instant pot and close the lid. Cook the spanakopita for 50 minutes on manual (high pressure). Then make a quick pressure release. Cool the cooked meal to room temperature and slice.

Nutrition: calories 319, fat 27.5, fiber 4.1, carbs 7.8, protein 12.9

Cheesy Radish Spread

Preparation time: 10 minutes

Cooking time: 10 minutes

Servings: 4

Ingredients:

- 2 cups radishes, sliced

- 4 ounces cream cheese, soft

- 1 cup cheddar cheese, grated

- ½ cup chicken stock

- ½ cup coconut cream

- A pinch of salt and black pepper

- 2 shallots, minced

- 1 teaspoon sweet paprika

Directions:

In your instant pot, combine all the ingredients, stir, put the lid on and cook on High for 12 minutes. Release the pressure naturally for 10 minutes, blend everything using an immersion blender, divide into bowls and serve.

Nutrition: calories 294, fat 20.6, fiber 1.8, carbs 5.4, protein 10.4

Conclusion

The immediate pot is such an innovative and futuristic food preparation tool. It has actually gotten many followers all over the globe. The immediate pot permits you to prepare delicious dishes for all your family in a matter of mins as well as with minimal effort. The best feature of the instantaneous pot is that you do not need to be a professional cook to make tasty culinary banquets. You simply require the right components and also the right directions. That's exactly how you'll get the best instant pot meals.

This fantastic culinary overview you have actually simply discovered is more than a straightforward immediate pot food preparation journal. It is a Ketogenic immediate pot dishes collection you will locate extremely helpful. The Ketogenic diet plan will provide you the power boost you need, it will make you lose the extra weight and also it will certainly improve your total wellness in a matter of days. This collection includes the most effective Ketogenic split second pot meals you can prepare in the convenience of your very own house. All these meals are so flavorful and distinctive as well as they all taste unbelievable.

So, if you are complying with a Ketogenic diet regimen and you have an instantaneous pot, get your very own duplicate of this recipe book as well as begin your Ketogenic culinary experience. Prepare the best Ketogenic immediate pot meals and also enjoy them all!

CPSIA information can be obtained
at www.ICGtesting.com
Printed in the USA
BVHW061031250521
608096BV00011B/1690